POWER UP YOUR BRAIN
Five Simple Strategies

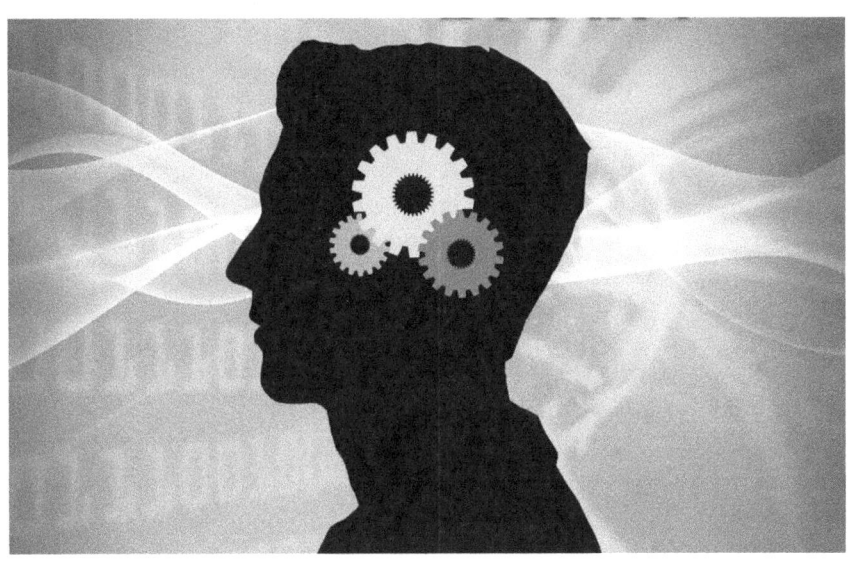

By J. J. Jackson

www.HowToImproveBrainPower.org

Power Up Your Brain
Five Simple Strategies
(c)2012, Blurtigo Holdings, LLC

Printed in United States of America

This book is dedicated to my children

Whitney, Brooke, Bryce, and Brock

*Thank you for listening to my dream of being
a published author for so many years.
It has finally become a reality*

Table of Contents

Introduction

Power Up Your Brain – Five Simple Strategies was written for everyone who wants to build and sustain a healthy brain regardless of age. It is my intention to introduce powerful strategies to you (some of them potentially life-changing) that will contribute to strong cognitive ability and memory power for a lifetime.

Not so long ago I realized that my brain was not functioning as well as it had in the past. In seemed that more and more I was struggling to remember where I had left my purse, my glasses, the grocery list I had just written, and so on.

At first, I joked about having "senior moments." After a while it began to wear on me, especially when I noticed that I was not processing information as quickly as I had in the past. My thinking was sluggish and I was losing my mental agility. I felt as if my brain were suddenly betraying me by not functioning at the level that it always had. That is when I decided to do something about it.

I was sure there was nothing wrong with my brain physiologically (even had a complete physical to make sure), but something was definitely off.

I thought about it long and hard and decided that I needed to find ways to boost my brain power back to earlier levels. I was sure that since there are many things that can be done to strengthen the structural muscles of the body; surely there must be things that could be done to strengthen the brain.

I set out to create my own brain fitness plan that would sharpen my thinking skills and improve my memory. I started seriously researching the principles of brain boosting and how to increase brain power and memory. The actions I needed to take began to fall into place and the plan took form.

As I developed and implemented the plan little by little, my brain power improved! The forgetfulness began to disappear and my brain started to regain its youthful agility.

I am now convinced that brain power and functionality have nothing to do with age; BUT . . . they are greatly impacted by lifestyle, which often becomes less disciplined as the years go by. If you are willing to learn the strategies and take action, you can easily keep your brain healthy and strong as you age.

The brain fitness strategies offered in this book were integral to my personal journey toward building a healthier brain. My goal in writing this book is to share with you exactly how I regained my mental agility, creativity, and the ability to recall anything in an instant.

In your twenties and thirties, you do not think about these amazing mental abilities because they are so natural and part of the gift of youth. But, as time goes by, it becomes important to be more aware, to pay attention to how your brain is functioning, and to do whatever is necessary to ensure that your mental abilities stay sharp throughout your life.

If you would like to improve your memory and boost your brain power, beginning today, you have made a wise first step in purchasing this book. You no longer need to worry or feel anxious about losing your mental acuity, because I am offering you ways to improve your brain power without drugs or expensive therapy.

There are three steps that must be taken to start this journey, so let's begin . . .

Step One: Make Brain Power a Priority

It takes a sincere desire to make the necessary changes in your lifestyle, coupled with implementation of daily action steps that will create and sustain the positive effects of the strategies that you choose.

If I were to tell you that there is one *surefire* way to boost your brain power, I would be misleading you – because the fact of the matter is that the human brain can be boosted and stimulated in so many ways that it is actually difficult to pick only a few strategies – there are simply so many of them!

Brain boosting should be part of your daily routine, much like bodybuilding. Your brain needs the proper food, adequate rest and regular workouts to get the results that you want. The results will be equivalent to the amount of effort that you put into the process.

Step Two: Read the Book

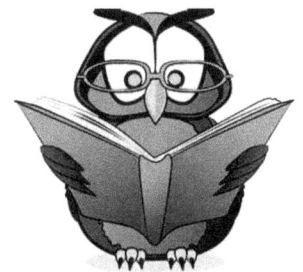

I recommend that you read straight through the book first, taking notes on the sections that you want to revisit. As you read, choose at least one action from each strategy as a starting point. Notice the ones that jump out at you as good possibilities.

The one exception to that suggestion is *The Basics.* All of the basics must be implemented if you are committed to the process; but, don't panic . . . there are choices within each basic category, such as food selection, types of exercise, etc.

Some strategies require more work than others. Your initial choices should be strategies that can be easily implemented. Give yourself a good chance for success. Then, add others one at a time until you have tried them all. You will eventually settle on several that work best for you – or, if you like all of them, switch them out for variety!

Step Three: Create a Plan of Action

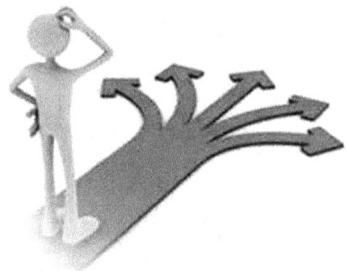

After you finish reading the book, create your plan of action. Be realistic and find a starting point that works. Do not fall into the trap of thinking that you have to do everything at once.

For example, when planning your steps for implementing *The Basics,* if you can't commit to buying brain-boosting supplements and the best organic foods available, a good first step would be to decrease your intake of fast food, energy drinks, and all foods with high quantities of sugar and fat.

When you are selecting action steps for *Brain Stimulation*, if you can't learn to play a musical instrument because of time and financial constraints, commit to reading for 15 minutes every night before going to sleep, or doing crossword puzzles during the "waiting" periods in your life.

Small doable steps are good. When those steps develop into habits, gradually introduce more steps. Eventually, you will have an excellent brain-boosting regimen integrated into your lifestyle. The results will be well worth the effort.

Keep your ACTION PLAN handy so you can review it regularly. Your journal would be a good choice, if you choose that as one of your action steps for managing stress.

I would also encourage you to track your results and record your progress in your journal to help you finalize your long-term action plan.

Remember - plans can, and should be changed. If you try something that simply doesn't work, try something else. BUT…be sure stay with a specific action step for at least 15 days before you discard it and try something different.

Everything in this book will improve your brain and memory power if you make a plan and stay with it. The results are up to you!

Good luck and enjoy the ride!

Strategy One: The Basics

The mind/body connection cannot be denied. They are two parts of a whole that cannot function separately. The state of the health of both parts defines the totality of what you can and cannot do – physically and mentally.

If you take care of one, you take care of the other. If your lifestyle harms one, it also harms the other. When the mind and body are fed, rested, exercised and properly challenged, you are unstoppable.

There are many things that can be done to increase your brain and memory power, but there are *three areas* of life that must be considered first because of their importance to your physical health and consequently, the health of your brain.

The problem is that two of them, food and rest, are so basic to your very existence and part of your everyday life that it is easy to forget how critical they are to brain health. As a result, habits often develop that can destroy your body and your magnificent brain a little bit at a time.

The third area, exercise, is something that happens naturally for children, but in adulthood a large number of people stop exercising completely, which also takes its toll on the body and the mind.

You are probably already aware of how these three things impact your physical health. But, let's look closely at how they also impact the brain. It is important to understand how "doing each of them right" will increase your brain power and "doing them wrong" will put you at risk for gradual diminished brain function and possibly at risk for much worse.

Basic #1: Feed Your Brain

*Let food be your medicine….*Hippocrates

The brain needs proper nutrition. The well-known adage, "You are what you eat," is true! Healthy eating habits are the **key** to your wellbeing.

Your diet must include all the necessary nutrients to nourish the 100 trillion cells in your body or those cells cannot function effectively! The food you eat affects everything: energy, sex drive, sleeping habits, and **the ability to think clearly.**

If your diet is mostly high-calorie junk food, fast foods, sugary sodas, and caffeine-filled energy drinks, your entire body will be affected, and the brain will no longer function at the levels of brilliance that it did when you were younger.

The brain controls and coordinates all the systems in the body, including the involuntary life-sustaining systems such as heart beat (cardio) and breathing (pulmonary). It also controls your physical actions (walk, talk, etc.) and the ability to interpret your surroundings through the five senses.

It filters and processes a massive amount of information and makes it possible for you to think, reason, dream and communicate with others. When the body does not receive proper nutrition, brain cells die and the brain's capacity to function properly is compromised, and your experience of life is diluted.

Included below is an in-depth discussion of 13 top food choices, a baker's dozen that you can incorporate into your diet to help your brain return to peak performance. While these brain foods were not chosen because they can physically heal the brain, each one contains nutrients that have been known to *enhance* the mental process and various brain functions.

It should be noted that *no food in existence* can improve your brain power in a few days. The natural approach to boosting your brain power requires patience and continuity. You will need to permanently integrate the suggestions into your daily lifestyle to obtain the long-term benefits.

If there are questions about any of the foods listed, e.g. allergies, sensitivities, etc., that could have a potential negative impact on your health, ***be sure to check with your doctor before incorporating them into your diet.***

My Top Thirteen Food Choices

The foods listed below are filled with nutrients that keep the mind healthy and help prevent degenerative brain disease. Because they are versatile in how they can be served, and easy on the palate, they can be incorporated easily into your diet without a lot of pain and struggle.

Most of them can be found at your local grocery store at reasonable cost. Three of my recommendations, Matcha, acai berries and wild salmon, are more difficult to find (and more expensive), but if you can find them and if they fit into your budget, they are excellent choices.

The foods are listed by categories: drinks, fruits and vegetables, whole grains, nuts and seeds, protein, spices, and chocolate (dessert).

Here we go . . .

Group One: Drinks

1. Coffee

For all you coffee lovers out there, coffee is NOT a vice! When it is pure, brewed coffee enjoyed in moderation (no more than two or three cups a day), it is a great way to start your day . . . and this is why. . .

Coffee beans are as awesome as cacao beans because quality, freshly brewed coffee *(minus the sugar/syrups, cream and other unhealthy things that people put into their customized concoctions)*, is actually a *super food* due to the number of nutrients it contains – including the caffeine. A word of caution on caffeine: Some people have sensitivities to caffeine or other contraindications that would make drinking coffee an unwise choice.

The coffee bean is also filled with anti-oxidants and for many Americans coffee is the primary (if not the only) source of anti-oxidants in their daily diet. So, keep up the good work, taking steps to modify the habit if you tend to overindulge.

Your morning coffee could very well be a small step toward preventing the onset of Alzheimer's disease, the insidious disease that affects the mental stability of a person by attacking the structure of the brain.

My suggestion would be to purchase a good coffee-maker or espresso maker (or both) and buy high-grade coffee beans that you grind and brew at home. Try different strengths and find the one that suits your personal taste.

For your daily dose of anti-oxidants, I recommend drinking a cup of good-quality black coffee or espresso (the best choice) in the morning. If you simply CANNOT drink coffee black, try *Stevia,* the natural herb sweetener, and unsweetened soy milk as a creamer. For a wonderful mid-afternoon pick-me-up switch to Matcha (be aware that it also contains caffeine), and end the day with a delicious cup of dark, hot chocolate (easy on the sugar – once again, *Stevia* is a perfect substitute). ENJOY!

2. Matcha

Matcha is made from stone-ground Japanese green tea leaves. It is NOT your common green tea neatly packaged in tea bags. You do not steep it and drink the flavored water; you drink/eat the "whole thing." It is a very different taste and takes some serious getting used to; but, it can be very addictive once you have acquired the taste.

There are actually three grades of Matcha – one for those new to the drink, another for those who know and love the drink, and the third which is to be used as an ingredient in sauces, lattes, etc. If you want to know more, visit: http://www.matchasource.com/about-matcha-s/19.htm.

There are some health benefits from most green teas, so I am not saying to stop drinking them, but consider the increased benefits from Matcha – a pure, ground green tea in concentrated, full-bodied form. You get straight, powerful doses of antioxidants, fiber, and vitamins A and C together with other important compounds such as L-theanine and *Epigallocatechin Gallate* (EGCG), which is known to have anti-cancer, anti-aging (another plus for the brain), as well as general health benefits. Be sure to stick with Japanese Matcha for the highest quality.

Because of the L-theanine, Matcha has long been used in Buddhist Monk ceremonies. It is both a stimulant and relaxant. The monks routinely drink it to stay calm, focused and awake during long 10-12 hour meditations. Imagine having the ability to put that kind of focus and prolonged energy into *your own work*. Your productivity could increase by leaps and bounds!

A study in Japan some years ago showed that people who drank tea four to five times a day lived *significantly longer* compared to people who didn't. But, let's kick it up a notch, shall we? If you really want to improve your brain power, you need to invest in something more potent than commercial green teabags.

Matcha is one of the life-changing habits I mentioned in the introduction. Are you willing to take action on this one?

Group Two: Fruits and Vegetables

3. Berries

Berries are full of anti-oxidants that are great for boosting brain power and reversing the effects of ageing. They are often called the "super fruits" and are particularly good for improving memory and recall.

The two berries I want to encourage you to include in your new *brain food diet* are the acai berry from Central and South America and the more well-known blueberry.

The acai berry contains the highest level of natural antioxidants of all commercially available berries. It also contains high levels of *protein, essential fatty acids, minerals, vitamins, and dietary fiber*. Because of its unusual nutrient profile, it is an excellent brain food.

To get the full benefits of the acai berry, I suggest that you buy them fresh or freeze-dried. You can also buy acai berry juice and powder. Please, be cautious about the numerous pills and products on the market that promote the health benefits of the berry. Read the labels carefully and do your homework before purchasing them. Be sure that you are not buying a product that is overly processed and lacking in any real health benefits.

You will also want to buy the more common and equally brain-healthy fruit: the blueberry – also known as the "brain berry."

A recent study by the USDA and Tufts University found that eating fresh or flash frozen blueberries on a daily basis may slow and even reverse age-related declines in the areas of the brain that control motor function, balance, and coordination, as well as improve short-term memory loss.

Blueberries are an easy, portable snack food, excellent on cottage cheese or Greek yoghurt, and adding fresh blueberries to whole-wheat pancakes, or hot oatmeal is a tasty, healthy way to eat more of this amazing fruit. Be careful with bakery items and mixes that include the berry because you could also be eating high levels of white flour, table sugar, and fat.

Since blueberries are available year-round in the produce section of most supermarkets, why not make a habit of eating them every day? A cup of blueberries a day is like downing nature's own brand of multivitamins and one of the best anti-oxidants around.

4. Apples

An apple a day keeps the doctor away . . . trite, but true when applied to a healthy brain. Recent research conducted at both the University of Massachusetts and Cornell University has shown that apples can help protect cognitive decline that accompanies ageing and can protect the brain from the type of damage that triggers Alzheimer's and Parkinson's.

A wide variety of fresh apples is available year round; so, pick your favorites and enjoy this crunchy, juicy treat every day. There is always delicious apple juice that can be enjoyed at breakfast or as a mid-afternoon pick-me-up. This is one of the easier ways to eat well for a healthier brain.

5. Avocados

Avocados are almost as good as blueberries in promoting brain health, and their value is often overlooked. They are rich with nutrients that improve memory, increase the ability to concentrate, and improve blood flow which results in lower blood pressure and decreases the risk of stroke.

Even though avocados are a fatty fruit that is high in calories, the fat is monounsaturated, the healthy fat, and a serving of one-quarter to one-half an avocado each day provides benefits to the heart and brain that are well worth the calories. Eat them fresh, and eat them often! Viva la guacamole!

6. Green Leafy Vegetables & Tomatoes

Everyone has been told, "Eat your vegetables. They are good for you!" As much as you may have dreaded hearing those words as a child, they are not hollow! Vegetables, especially all of the green leafy ones, are good for you, particularly for the brain!

They are rich in Vitamin B, which helps protect against cognitive decline as you get older. Broccoli should be one of your top choices because it also contains Vitamin K, another important vitamin that keeps the brain clear and sharp.

The versatile tomato can be used in so many dishes that people don't even notice them anymore; however, did you know that tomatoes are rich in a substance called lycopene?

Lycopene is a powerful antioxidant that has been shown to protect the brain by helping to prevent degenerative conditions like dementia. In addition to lycopene, a single tomato contains a long list of important vitamins, all important to brain health. So, with a little modification, let's try this again . . .

Eat your vegetables. They are good for your brain!"

Group Three: Whole Grains, Nuts & Seeds

7. Whole Grains

The reason for this particular recommendation is that whole grain foods contain B vitamins (particularly vitamin B6, which contains thiamine) and folate. Recent studies have shown that if you increase your intake of foods rich in these essential nutrients, your recall memory will improve.

All whole grain foods such as whole wheat, bran, brown rice, whole-grain breads, oatmeal, barley, and so on, are known to increase blood flow to the brain, which is vital for high-level brain function.

If you enjoy eating breads and pastas, I suggest that you make a complete switch to whole-grain products so you take advantage of better health benefits as you enjoy your macaroni or spaghetti at home. Anything that is whole grain is a good choice – go for it!

8. Nuts and Seeds

Looking for a source of Omega-3 fatty acids other than fish to help your brain function more efficiently? Well, look no more! Fresh, raw refrigerated walnuts and chia seeds are excellent alternatives and both can be easily incorporated into your diet in a multitude of ways. In addition to Omega 3 fatty acids, they are full of Omega-6 fatty acids, which work as a natural antidepressant.

Nuts and seeds are hailed as a great source of nutrients that help with everything from insomnia to memory loss because in addition to the fatty acids already mentioned, they contain folate, minerals, vitamin E and vitamin B6 – all nutrients that enhance clarity of thought. The zinc found in a small handful of pumpkin seeds everyday will go along way toward strengthening your memory and recall.

You can choose from raw or dry roasted peanuts, almonds, pecans, flax seeds and sunflower seeds – to name a few. There are nuts and seeds for every palate. In addition to being an exceptionally healthy snack food because they are portable and do not need refrigeration, they are an excellent ingredient that adds texture, flavor and character to everything from salad to dessert.

Group Four: Oily Fish

9. Wild Salmon

If you want to get the greatest benefits of eating fish, it would be wise to put forth the effort to find *wild salmon,* which unfortunately, is getting harder and harder to do. It is one of the healthier foods, as well as the best fish you can eat and is a *safer* choice than farmed salmon. Wild salmon is not filled with chemical additives, artificial coloring, preservatives, pesticides, growth hormones, and antibiotics.

Farmed salmon (like most farmed sources of meat) are fatty because they have not been able to *age* like wild salmon. Wild salmon have time to grow and plenty of space to move around in order to develop darker muscle tissue and higher levels of Omega 3 fatty acids.

Wild salmon is not only rich in Omega 3 acids, which are necessary for optimum heart and brain health – especially as you age - it is also rich in protein and amino acids. Studies show that it helps to keep your cardiovascular system working at optimum level and can potentially help reduce the risk of Alzheimer's disease.

Group Five: Other Protein

10. Eggs

Eggs (in moderation – no more than one or two a day) are critical to maintaining a healthy brain. They contain vitamin B12 and lecithin, which help prevent brain shrinkage, which is often seen in Alzheimer patients. Eggs also contain Omega 3 fatty acids and are high in choline, an important building block of brain cells.

Eating eggs for breakfast helps reboot your body and your brain as a much-needed energy source after eight to ten hours without food. The nutrients in eggs help with concentration, memory recall and problem-solving capabilities – all important functions of the brain.

11. Lentils

Lentils are a particularly excellent choice for vegetarians. They are high in protein, dietary fiber, and anti-oxidants. They are full of iron and contain brain-friendly phytonutrients, which aid in the prevention of cell damage. Iron is a critical nutrient that increases oxygen flow to the brain and fights fatigue – the biggest obstacle to concentration.

These small, delicious beans cook up quickly in soups and stews without a long initial soaking. They can be served alone as the main dish or cooked with lean meat and other vegetables for an all-in-one, easy meal. Spice up the lentils with curry, another of our top 13 brain foods, and you have a powerhouse dish that will feed your brain with a host of important nutrients.

Group Six: Spices and Garlic

12. Curcumin & Garlic

Curcumin, the ultimate brain spice, is the primary compound in Turmeric, a root native to Indonesia and India. Turmeric can be used fresh or dried on salads, vegetables, meat and seafood. It is also used as the base of most curry powder, a key ingredient in many types of Indian dishes.

Both turmeric and curry are aromatic, spicy, delicious and easy to find. There is no reason not to include one or both in your diet. They not only spice up your food, but also spice up your brain. Because curcumin is full of anti-oxidants, it fights against brain aging and sustains cognitive function as you age physically. It guards against Dementia, Alzheimer's and Parkinson's disease – all insidious diseases of the brain.

If spicy foods are a problem for you, be assured that you do not have to force feed it to yourself every day – a small serving once a month will produce important benefits to your brain.

Garlic, a staple ingredient in many ethnic foods, has been proven to prevent age-related loss of cognitive functions, particularly age-related memory disorders. This is a simple add to many dishes. Some people choose to eat it alone, either raw or baked. Find your pleasure.

Group Seven: Dark Chocolate

13. Cacao

The well-loved chocolate bar is partially derived from the cacao bean, which contains important nutrients. However, I do not recommend that you eat copious amounts of chocolate candy just so you can get the cacao content. Delicious as it may be, most chocolate bars contain very low levels of the cacao bean and are filled with sugar and milk fat. If you MUST eat chocolate candy, be sure to choose high-quality dark-chocolate with a cacao content of 75% or higher.

Current research has suggested that cacao (not processed chocolate products) is actually an all-around health ranger that protects not only a person's cognitive function but also the skin and heart. Cacao is rich in the anti-oxidant, known as flavonols, which are necessary for optimum health because they increase blood flow to the brain. Quality dark chocolate is rich in flavonols.

Be aware that cacao itself is *not* sweet and buttery like most of the chocolate candy you know and love. It is actually bitter. The easiest way to get the benefits of this age-old health food is to mix high-quality cacao powder into any of your existing beverages (such as coffee). To cut the bitter taste, add a little natural sweetener such as *Stevia*, made from a South American herb, and a dash of cinnamon. Enjoy this nutrient-rich drink (hot or cold) and happily remember that the tasty drink is boosting your brain power at the same time!

To conclude this section, below are general guidelines for selecting foods to feed your brain and foods to avoid:

Brain-boosting Foods	Brain-draining Foods
Organic foods	Overly-processed foods
Whole Grains & Brown Rice	Greasy foods
Fresh Fruits & Vegetables	Sugar & Sugary Foods
Nuts & Seeds	White Flour
Oily Fish & Oysters	Saturated Fat
Lean Beef	Hydrogenated Fat
Chicken & Turkey	Fast Foods
Milk & Yoghurt	Artificial Flavoring & Coloring
Soybeans	Artificial Sweeteners
Pure Nut Butters	Sodas (Regular & Diet)
Legumes (beans)	Chips, Cheetos, etc.
Wheat Germ	Energy Drinks(Red Bull, etc.)
Brewer's Yeast	Cereal Bars & Donuts, etc.
Flaxseed Oil	Alcohol & Nicotine

Take Natural Brain Boosting Supplements

Since many brain boosting supplements are available, it would be wise to spend some time researching them from the actual product websites. Below are some suggestions that you may want to check out.

Gingko biloba has long been revered as a medicinal wonder because of the multiple conditions that people report it could cure. I am not saying that gingko biloba is an actual cure for anything, *but* for a long period of time, people have been drinking tea infused with this root to improve concentration and thinking.

If you're not allergic to it, then by all means, find a gingko biloba supplement that works for you. Studies have shown that gingko biloba can actually increase the brain's blood supply by increasing the blood flow to this organ.

Since gingko biloba is widely cultivated, it is inexpensive compared to other supplements. It will not leave a big dent in your monthly budget. The dosage for most gingko biloba supplements is only to 1 to 2 tablets or capsules a day.

As I have already mentioned earlier, more blood to the brain literally means more oxygen – and oxygen is *brain food.* The brain can't get enough of it because it is constantly firing chemical and electrical signals throughout the body to keep everything functioning normally.

St. John's Wort has been around for more than 10 years, and although it doesn't directly help boost your brain power, it has been used by many people suffering from clinical depression. The indirect effect on the brain is that a lighter, positive outlook always helps you think more clearly.

Omega-3 fatty acids improve memory, learning ability, and may also prevent depression, mood disorders, schizophrenia, and dementia. A large percentage of the gray matter in the brain is made up Omega-3 fatty acids. These help make brain cells more fluid and in turn, improve communication between brain cells. DHA also seems to slow down the build up of a protein that forms neurofibrillary tangle in the brain, a contributing factor in Alzheimer's disease.

As mentioned earlier, one of the best food sources for Omega-3 is oily fish, particularly wild salmon, and there are other options. Fresh, raw refrigerated walnuts and chia seeds are excellent alternatives and both can be easily incorporated into your diet in a multitude of ways. In addition to Omega 3 fatty acids, they are full of Omega-6 fatty acids, which work as a natural antidepressant.

As you can see, Omega-3 is available in a number of foods, but if you choose to take it in capsule form, the recommended dose via food and/or supplements is 1,000 to 3,000 milligrams daily

Below are four additional supplements that you may want to consider. These four are often found in combination supplement capsules or tablets.

1. **Nattokinase** (from soybeans) helps with blood flow in the body – including the brain, which is critical for lifelong mental acuity.

2. **Alpha Lipoic acid** (aLa) is one of the best antioxidants for the brain.

3. **Phosphatidyl Serine** (PS) helps with memory recall, especially numbers, names and faces, etc.

4. **Acetyl-L-Carnitine** helps brain produce a vital neurotransmitter and is often used in the treatment of Alzheimer's disease.

Herbal supplements are not always safe just because they have been derived primarily from plants. Many herbal plants are quite potent. There can be side effects, sensitivities and possible negative interactions with medications that you are taking. *It is vital that you always consult with your doctor before adding supplements of any kind to your diet.*

Basic #2: Get Adequate Rest

Need I say more? Rest is absolutely essential to good health. People brag that they feel perfectly rested after only four or five hours of sleep each night; but, they aren't and probably don't even realize it!

Lack of adequate sleep not only affects your brain function (recall, retention, concentration, etc.) but also negatively impacts your general health. In addition to taking a toll on your brain power, lack of adequate rest increases the risk for cancer, stroke and heart attacks.

Most people who are suffering from memory-related problems are often physically fine. They may be suffering from sleep deprivation, which leaves the mind and body exhausted and unable to function properly. If your job and family responsibilities make seven to eight hours of sleep almost impossible, power naps become essential to your health.

Learn to Power Nap

A power nap right after lunch can give you a significant recharge. The longer the nap, the better; but, even 20 minutes will make you more efficient and alert. Longer naps boost energy and enhance creativity. And, a 60- to 90-minute nap (should you be so lucky) is ideal for increasing brain function.

The benefits of power naps add up during the week, and your whole body (including your brain) will appreciate the fact that you are setting aside even short periods of time for rejuvenation.

Finding time for power naps can be a simple way of solving your challenge to get enough rest at night, or at least, alleviate it to some degree. The place you nap is not important (cars are very good), but taking the nap is important . . . and make them as long as possible.

One final note regarding the importance of resting the mind and body: sacrificing adequate rest for "the job" is never a wise choice. Work is important because it gives direction to your life and provides the basic physical necessities for daily living. But work should *never* be allowed to be the cause of complete mental and/or physical exhaustion, which puts your health at risk. No job is worth it! If you are in that position, it may be time to re-evaluate!

Basic #3: Exercise Regularly

Many people have a daily exercise regimen. Some center around cardiovascular and heart pumping exercises, others center on weight training, others walk/run several miles a day, and so on. Kudos go out to everyone who is disciplined enough to take care of their body in this way.

The best part about regular exercise is that it not only strengthens the physical body, it also increases brain power! In fact, exercise has proven repeatedly that it is an efficient and natural way to improve the mind's ability to process information quickly.

Physical exercise is one of the building blocks of an alert and powerful mind. You may have learned in high school biology that exercise gets the heart pumping, increases circulation by widening the arteries, and increases the flow of oxygen to the brain – all of which causes the brain to function more effectively.

Exercise also increases the release of endorphins, morphine-like molecules, that impact the way the neurotransmitters operate – and they make you feel good. Voilà - A healthier, (happier), more efficient brain.

Using junk food, energy drinks, drugs or alcohol as stimulants to get the creative juices flowing (or to feel better) may work in the short-term, but the ultimate cost you pay in damage to your body through addiction, physical deterioration, and loss of brain cells is NOT worth it. Going for a run, walking on the treadmill, or dancing in your living room are much better choices to clear the head and spark creativity!

An exercise routine does not mean you have to sign up for a gym membership and lift heavy weights like professional bodybuilders. The best workouts will be something you enjoy doing and can look forward to because of the way it makes you feel.

Don't buy into the "no pain – no gain" philosophy. That statement is true to a point. You do have to stretch yourself beyond what is comfortable in order to reap the full benefits, but you don't have to hurt yourself.

Start slow and build up. Set small, reachable goals and when you are ready, take it up to the next level. The truth of the matter is that even a 20 minute semi-brisk walk three times a week with a friend can be an excellent choice.

There are as many types of physical activities as there are days in a year (perhaps even more!), so get out there and find one (or two, or three) that you enjoy. It won't be long until your body will begin to crave the exercise when you miss a day. Physical fitness definitely contributes to mental fitness, no matter what your age.

Since all three of *The Basics* directly impact the cardio-pulmonary system, there is one addendum that must be included …

Monitor and Manage Blood Pressure

Recent studies have shown that older adults who are suffering from high blood pressure are more at risk for declining cognitive performance than individuals who are managing their condition, either through medication or natural blood pressure control methods (i.e. meditation, diet modification, etc.). This decline has always been attributed to ageing, but doctors now believe it is often the result of long-term hypertension.

If you are in your twenties or thirties, high blood pressure is especially serious because the effects of high blood pressure on your cognitive performance over time are cumulative.

Hypertension, so often ignored or even undiagnosed, can ultimately take your life. In the meantime, it will reap havoc with your ability to concentrate, your memory, and your ability to reason and make decisions.

Have your blood pressure checked regularly. If it has been a while – have it checked soon. If it is elevated, do whatever you need to do to get it down to an acceptable level. The health of your heart and your brain depend on it!

Strategy Two: Stress Management

Stress is a natural physiological response of the body to danger or pressure that produces chemicals resulting in extra energy and strength for protection (flight or fight).

Life is never stress free. Everyone deals with it from time to time. Some people are able to move in and out of it without problems because they have learned techniques that allow them to manage it effectively. Other people are not so lucky. Which are you?

The four most common stressors are:

1. Physical danger

2. Environmental and external factors (noise, crowds, negative voices, work pressures)

3. Being overwhelmed, exhausted or overworked (feeling that life is out-of-control)

4. Internal pressure to perform/succeed or to control the uncontrollable

Stressors that come from life changes cannot be avoided, such as financial struggles, death of family members or friends, the holidays, pregnancy, parenthood, and divorce. It is critical to learn to manage these unavoidable stressors and find ways to remove or avoid other stressors whenever possible.

Manage Stress or Pay the Price

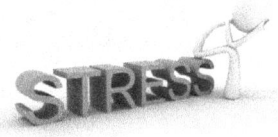

Long-term, unmanaged stress affects both the mind and the body, creating fatigue, illness and an inability to concentrate and think clearly. High, sustained levels of stress can actually cause you to feel like you are going to explode or break down from the mounting pressure.

Many people deal with heavy levels of stress on a daily basis, but do not recognize the problem signs and are unaware of the health threat for both mind and body. Let's take a quick look at some of the danger signals.

Long-term stress can affect you physically: your appetite – eating too much or not enough; sleeping patterns – sleeping too much or too little resulting in sleep deprivation; your immune system - making you susceptible to colds, asthma, ulcers, migraines, etc.; your sex drive/performance; and your stamina – creating chronic fatigue.

It also affects you mentally, which can be manifested by feelings of anxiety, constant worry, panic attacks; feeling out of control and confused; development of addictions; neglect of personal hygiene, work and family responsibilities; unwarranted fears of physical illness or natural disasters.

It is not uncommon to experience one or two of the above problems from time to time without cause for concern. But, if the number increases and they tend to be habitual, you are probably dealing with more stress than you realize. If that happens, you must find ways to identify and deal with the stressors in order to protect your mental and physical health.

Take Steps to Manage Your Stress

We have already discussed the importance of a good diet, adequate rest and regular exercise. When any of these areas are lacking or out of control, it will add stress to your mind and body. Consequently, it stands to reason that when those three things are well covered, they will help alleviate stress.

In addition to the basics, it is critical to implement other strategies to help eliminate stress – or at least, manage it well.

The first step is to look closely at your life – what is causing the pressure? Are the stressors external or internal? (See the four most common sources of stress described above).

Don't lie to yourself or quickly skim over problems. If something is bothering you, acknowledge that it is and try to figure out *why* it is bothering you. When you can identify what is causing the stress, and hopefully why, you have a better chance of figuring out what to do about it.

1. Seriously consider perceived obligations

- Do you try to be superman (or woman), feeling responsible to be all things, to all people, at all times?
- Have you adopted the role of caretaker to friends and family, believing that you must be available to listen to and to fix their problems?
- Are you working all the time to buy things for yourself and your family that everyone (including you) may be very happy living without?
- Are you allowing the little things to control the big things? What are your priorities – really?
- Do you ever make your personal wellbeing a priority?

2. Figure out what you can change (or not)

- Change what you can change; and change your attitude and typical responses to the things that you cannot change.
- *Always keep in mind that you cannot control anyone's attitude or behavior <u>except your own</u>, so stop trying!*
- Change your own (comfortable) attitudes and behavior patterns that do not work. This is particularly important in challenging relationships and the work environment.

3. Put difficult relationships and situations in perspective

- Watch the intensity of your reactions to people and situations. Are you interpreting them in such a way that they are more stressful than they need to be?
- Develop tools that help you to *act rather than react.* Train yourself to always pause and take a breath before responding. If you feel like you are going to lose it, walk away.
- Take time to examine what is really going on for you emotionally that may be causing the intensity of your reaction. This can help diffuse the strength of what you are feeling and allow you to deal with the person or situation in a more effective way. And – most important, it will help ease the stress that you are putting on yourself.

4. Manage your time better

- Be clear about your priorities and take care of the top ones first.

- Learn to say NO. Making promises that you cannot keep without stressing yourself out, serves no one, especially not you.
- Be willing to let secondary things go without worrying about them. Accept the fact that you only have so many hours in each day.
- Create a schedule with blocks of time for the priorities.
- Work on the most important and demanding things during your most productive hours.
- Schedule a little personal time each day – to power nap, meditate, take a luxurious bath or long, hot shower – be good to yourself.

5. Avoid stuffing your emotions!

- Let yourself laugh, cry, scream, yell, or pound something (preferably a pillow, grass, sand – not the wall). Do whatever you need to do, probably in private is the best choice. But, if emotions erupt in public, excuse yourself and let it rip. This is nature's way of releasing stress. Don't beat yourself up afterward!
- You must find a safe and sane way to release your emotions (this applies to both men and women) When you continually stuff them, you are endangering your own health and possibly the well being of others around you.
- Stuffed emotions eventually come out – either in the form of a physical illness, a mental break down, or incredible explosions of anger on anyone who happens to be around – including your children (innocent bystanders.
- Don't set yourself or your family up for these consequences.

6. BREATHE and use quick tension-release exercises

- There is a saying, "Breathe like a Buddha." Find out what this means and try it.
- Anthony Robbins also has some great breathing exercises in his book, *The Giant Within*.
- Relaxing sounds simple, but can be quite difficult for some people. Individuals, who carry tension in their neck and shoulders, may find quick tension-relieving exercises for those areas very helpful. Even simple stretching exercises for the neck, shoulders, arms and back can help a lot.
- Check the Internet – there are dozens of breathing exercises and quick upper body relaxation techniques that you can learn – and they work!
- Find a few that work for you and do them several times a day. I promise they will give you much needed breaks, which will relieve stress and refresh your mind.

The next five action steps are not only excellent brain boosters, they also tie in closely to some of the actions listed above for relieving stress. In other words, you are getting double benefit when you use them.

For instance, the first one, map mapping is a wonderful tool to help organize your life, or segments of your life, which can help you with managing your time and making commitments.

Try Mind Mapping

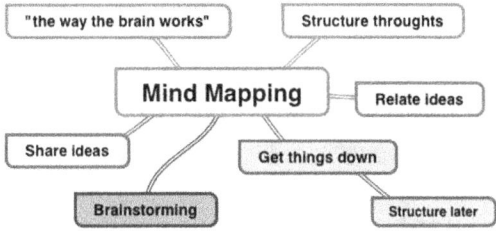

Map mapping works the way your brain works. The process is both analytical and creative and engages both sides of your brain, which makes it a great brain-stimulating exercise.

It gets everything down on paper, facilitates brainstorming and sharing ideas, structures thoughts, relates ideas, and allows structuring of a plan to move forward.

It is best to create your mind map by hand either on paper or on a large board. If you want to buy something to improve your mind mapping experience, I recommend a large sketch pad. It is important to have plenty of paper available so you do not feel limited on space. A notebook is another smaller, less-costly option and also works well. It just takes more pages.

Since I hope that you will be creating mind maps later on, either for your personal use or for your work, buying a thick sketch book would be worth it. The best thing about this activity is that you can easily take your pad or notebook with you wherever you go and use "waiting times" to work on the map.

If you like technology (i.e. tablet computers), there are sketching software programs for mind maps, but the experience will be a little subdued because you won't have the same freedom that you have when you create a mind map manually.

Some people think of mind maps as really crazy, loopy maps of ideas and words. At the outset, a mind map *may* look crazy to someone, but only because it is not his or her mind map. In short, mind maps are personal expressions that tend to make sense only to their creators.

You can certainly share mind maps with anyone you like, but that doesn't mean your audience will automatically understand your map, because no two people think alike. What makes perfect sense to you may be confusing and utterly baffling to the person across the table.

When you are ready to create your very first mind map, this is how you do it:

1. Choose one thing that you want to plan or map out. It can be a story that you've always wanted to write, your new leadership project for school, or a plan to make a million dollars in ten years. It doesn't matter what it is. All you need a viable starting point.

2. Break down the idea into two or three "big ideas." For example, if you want to make a million dollars, your big ideas may include 1) Creating unique products that people love. 2) Producing those products. 3) Marketing the products.

    This is just a sample starting point. Don't work about how many "big ideas" you have at first. You can have one or twenty-five. It doesn't matter. You can expand on your plan indefinitely using your mind map.

3. Start your map in the middle of the page (landscape orientation) with a word or two words in the center that describes the purpose of the map – the "project" or "goal."

4. Connect each of the first few big ideas to the center with colorful lines, and start expanding them. After the

first level of expansion, you can start creating more big idea branches on the map. Don't worry, the ideas will come. Once your brain is engaged, the creative juices start flowing and ideas will pop. Suspend judgment and capture them with flair. The main thing is to have fun with this process.

5.   Keep your topic labels simple, only one or two words. Even better, use pictures!

6.   If one page isn't enough, move on to the next page. (That is the beauty of having a large sketch pad – plus the larger maps are easier to read!).

7.   Don't be afraid to use adequate spacing and long, curving lines to distinctly separate large groups of ideas from one another.

8.   If one idea leads to another, clearly connect those two ideas together. In the end, you will have a mind map that looks exactly like the nerve cells in the brain.

9.   Use bold colors, wild symbols, and funny stick figures. Restraint is not allowed! The more flamboyant you are, the more creative your mind becomes!

10.   Vary the thickness, length, and colors when drawing the connecting lines. Find unique ways to emphasize important points. The more relaxed you are and the more fun you have, the more engaged your mind will be!

Write Things Down

Putting your thoughts down on paper (journaling) is an excellent tool for managing stress and boosting brain power in general.

If you want to improve your memory and your recall, writing things down is a surefire way to increase this brain function. When you record information, your thoughts, ideas, events, etc., the brain builds the neurons necessary for instant recall when you want or need it.

There are many types of journaling, each of which requires a different focus and level of concentration. The one thing the types have in common is that they all stimulate the brain and tap into pockets of emotion that generate powerful feelings.

Feelings need to be recognized, experienced and released, which journaling can help you do. Stuffing your feelings or denying that emotions exist can cause relentless mental anguish and unnecessary stress on your mind and body.

When you empty your mind on paper, it releases the tension that results from running things over and over in your mind, better known as worry.

Constant worry takes its toll on the mind, interferes with the ability to think clearly and hampers concentration. The release of tension that comes from writing down your thoughts can be mentally freeing and tends to relax both the mind and the body.

Journaling can also be helpful if your thinking patterns are typically random and disorganized, or if you have trouble making decisions.

When the mind is forced to sort through all the known information about whatever is bothering you and has to work hard to organize it enough for you to put the words on paper, it gets an excellent workout. That is exactly what it needs to stay agile and sharp – and it should happen as often as possible.

Journaling is one of the best ways to organize and clarify your thoughts. Sometimes total clarity on a particular problem takes several journal entries. But, if you stay with it, clarity will come.

Journaling is also an exceptional form of self-expression and provides moments of quiet reflection on your life experiences – good and bad. It is most effective if you can relax and let the mind take you where it will. Free-flow writing can be a remarkably pleasurable experience.

There are many ways to journal. By hand, which is my preference, but you can also journal on your computer. There is even software available to help you. Or, if you want to share your thoughts publicly – start a blog! You may want to try both private and public journaling. They each have their place and serve very different purposes. Both are great stimulants for the mind

If you feel your thoughts belong only to you, and you enjoy the solitude and peace that a regular journal provides, then stick with a paper journal or notebook.

Journaling should be all about *you.* The activity should *please YOU – no one else.* Don't focus on anything except recording the words. Don't worry about perfect handwriting, spelling, grammar, etc.; but, I would encourage you to make it legible, because at some point you will probably want to read it.

This activity should not be a burden and does not have to be done every day. Write when you are so inclined, when something happens, when life throws you an unexpected curve, when you are feeling great emotion or are struggling with a problem.

If you enjoy the process, I encourage you to make it part of your routine – daily or weekly are both good choices.

If you dread doing it or find it unpleasant for any reason, DON'T do it. Journaling is not for everyone and may not be the best option for you. But, if you enjoy it at all, even writing occasionally can be a lovely boost to the mind.

Journaling is easy, low/no cost, and no preparation needed. All you have to do is start writing.

Socialize Often

Humans are social beings. It is unfortunate that fast-paced lifestyles often prevent connections with others on a personal level. In fact, isolation is a stressor. Everyone needs a support system, including you, and you need to find time to go out and have fun with your friends.

Socializing has two main benefits that contribute to a healthy brain:

1. Regular social interaction challenges and stimulates the brain in ways that are simply not possible alone. When the brain is stimulated by great conversation and humorous exchanges that are accompanied by laughter, the neural network is expanded.

2. It reduces the risk factor for depression and other mental illnesses. People who live in relative isolation, with very little outside contact and do not participate in social activities are at a much higher risk for those problems.

Finally - spending time with friends and colleagues that you enjoy and who can take your mind of work and everything else you have to do can be a great stress reliever. You owe it to yourself to decompress in this way from time to time – and not just at the holidays. Having fun gives the brain a huge boost and makes you feel better all over.

Eliminate Negative External Voices

Negative external voices fall into the category of environmental stressors. This is one area that you can control, if you try, but it may require breaking some deeply ingrained habits.

If you feel compelled to watch the news every night and/or read several newspapers every day, I urge you to break the habit. Avoid any kind of news, except maybe the weather and sports. (I realize there are some things you simply cannot give up) The best choice would be to stop devouring negative stories/news from any source – including online.

Be selective about the information that you choose to fill your mind. Negative stories (voices) that are focused on the horrors of life, mistakes and limitations of others provide no value – and they are not good for you. The only thing they do is add stress to your life.

Choose to fill your mind with good things (actions, words, events, etc.) Seek out news that is joyful, uplifting and tell stories of lives well-lived.

Another source of negative voices that you should limit as much as possible is from people in your life - what they say *to* you and *about* you. You do not have to listen, you can walk away. If you are forced to listen, let the words pass quickly through your mind. Do not allow them to run rampant inside your brain. Those thoughts are wild, loose bullets that continue to do damage long after the initial impact.

By avoiding, or at least limiting negative external voices, you will enjoy life more because you will be internalizing only positive information. That choice helps to clear the mind, clarifies your thinking process, and builds pleasant memories that enhance your outlook on life and overall health of the brain.

Learn to Meditate

Meditation is the last action that connects directly to stress management. It combines physical and mental relaxation to achieve a state of physical calm and mental clarity.

Not so long ago, meditation was looked upon as strange and only practiced by a fringe element of society who studied and accepted Eastern Medicine.

Some believe that it may have originated accidentally in ancient times when people fell into a meditative states while watching the flames of their fires. Over many centuries it evolved into a structured practice used by mystics and monks throughout the Far East to gain an understanding of the mysteries of life.

Today, it is practiced around the world by people in all walks of life as a way to lower anxiety levels, to relax, to clear the mind and also to manage stress. The physical and mental health benefits are significant.

In the January 30, 2011 issue of *Psychiatry Research: Neuroimaging* researchers reported the meditation for 30 minutes a day for eight weeks has measurable changes in gray-matter density in parts of the brain associated with memory, sense of self, empathy, and stress.

There are also other current studies that indicate mindfulness meditation can be a powerful practice for individuals suffering from bi-polar and other mood disorders. Mindfulness meditation is focused on breathing and being in the moment. It helps the individuals to relax and, to push away troubling thoughts – something that could be helpful to most of us.

Advocates and long-time practitioners of meditation will tell you that everything positive that is said about meditation is true. Why not see for yourself? It is certainly worth trying.

If you cannot carve out a quiet time and space in your home, another option is to using a meditation center, where you can meditate undisturbed in a serene environment.

If you want to learn more, research it on the Web or pick up a good book on meditation from your local bookstore and see how it works for you.

I am sure you are going to be surprised with the results that will come overtime if you stay with it. Don't expect miracles. It is not necessarily easy, at least in the beginning because you may have no idea how to relax and empty your mind. It takes practice. Also, avoid blocking your progress by negative self-talk about the process. Look forward to improvement that will come, and give your brain time to adapt to this new, useful activity.

Strategy Three: Brain Stimulation

The brain is our most important organ – it is what makes us human. Yet, we often forget to take care of our brains as carefully as we take care of our physical bodies.

Without regular stimulation that comes from social interaction and challenges, brain functions deteriorate. It is common knowledge that if you don't use your muscles, they lose strength.

It is the same with the brain. If you don't use it all the time, its power will begin to diminish. It must be stimulated regularly in order to stay at peak performance levels.

Play Games

One of the easiest ways to stimulate the mind is through games. Some people think games are for children, and stop playing them when they become "adults." What a shame! There is a child in you that needs to come out and play often!

Any kind of game(s) will do – competitive sports such as tennis and basketball (which also include the physical exercise component, a two-for-one effort), board games, puzzles, and cards to name a few.

Be sure to keep social interaction as part of the mix. Invite friends and family over to play games as often as possible. If you are retired or have the time, find a community center that has regular game nights or join a Bridge club.

If none of those choices are available to you, video games are a good alternative. They can be can be played alone and still provide the much needed brain stimulation. They are better than nothing, but playing games with other people is SO much better. The stimulation is exponentially greater.

There are a wide variety of gaming consoles available: Kinect, Wii, PlayStation, Nintendo DS, PC games, etc. The important thing is that you find a way to play games.

Playing an hour a day is excellent, but don't overdo it. Playing video games all day and rarely doing anything else is not a good choice. This is a case where more is NOT better.

Do Puzzles

Some people love puzzles and some people hate them. They are purposefully designed to confound you, and sometimes take a lot of work to figure them out. That is exactly why they are great stimulant for your brain. Doing puzzles is an awesome way to increase your brain power.

When you work on crossword puzzles, Sudoku, and others, you are challenging your brain in ways that it is not typically challenged in every day life.

Puzzles force your brain to expend cognitive resources to help you be successful. The frustration that you feel when you seem to hit a brick wall is actually just your mind working tirelessly to solve the puzzle.

If your life is fairly normal, you must have chunks of time that you spend "waiting" for someone or some thing. Those forced waiting periods can be 10 minutes or two hours, depending on the situation. Rather than do nothing, make them productive by filling them with the great brain-boosting activity of solving puzzles.

Try keeping a New York Times Crossword Puzzle Book handy, or download puzzles onto your Smartphone. Since you probably never leave home without your phone, you will always be prepared.

Using those waiting periods to work on puzzles ensures that you will be engaging in this activity regularly – a very good thing. The more you do it, the greater the benefits. Five minutes here and five minutes there will add up – and your brain will thank you.

Read! Read! Read!

Find time in your life to read! If possible read a little everyday! With tablet computers and e-readers such as Kindle, it is no longer necessary to buy hardcopy books, although they are still my personal preference. There is something safe and familiar about holding a book in your hands and absorbing the words from each page, allowing yourself to be whisked into another world for a few moments in time . . . the great escape.

Books are one of the great mind stimulators. The written word can have a powerful impact on your emotions, often sending you into sensory overdrive. It can also challenge your reason and logic. A good book will stimulate both sides of your brain, sometimes leaving a lasting impression in its wake.

The brain benefits of reading are immense, which makes reading a great action step if you want to boost your mental prowess.

If you haven't picked up a good book in years, your reading is restricted to work-related topics, or you steal a few moments here or there to read on the Internet, it is time to make a change. Pay a visit to the local library or a good bookstore – or take advantage of some of the great book bargains that can be purchased through stores that recycle donated books. Two of my favorites are Bookman's and Savers. And . . . there are always the electronic stores, such as *The Kindle Store* on *Amazon*.

The type of book and the book source are not important - just start reading!

Learn Something New

Psychologists and therapists from related fields all agree that continuous learning is essential if you want to keep your mind robust and agile. Learning something new now and then is an excellent way to keep your brain agile and sharp!

Don't go out and take on a challenge that will overwhelm you and may quickly become discouraging. Start slowly and begin to develop the habit of seeking out new things to learn on a regular basis. Try something new everyday like driving a different route work to and/or from work, or introduce yourself to at least one new person at work every week – really get to know them.

Make a list of some of the things that you have always wanted to do and start doing them:

1. Take voice lessons or learn to play the piano.

2. Learn to speak Spanish, French, German.

3. Build a remote control truck and learn to race it.

4. Take a speed-reading course.

5. Volunteer at the library, the hospital, a soup kitchen, or a shelter for abused women.

   a. Learn all the ropes and be one of the best volunteers they have.

   b. Volunteering combines so many stimuli that any one of them would be a phenomenal choice.

6. Start an herb or flower garden in your yard.

7. Take an interior design course and redecorate your bedroom.

8. Learn how to frame pictures or create a bonsai tree.

9. You get the idea . . . start your own list and take action today!

Tickle Your Senses

The senses of hearing and sight are most commonly used to process the world around you. Those two senses do the job well, but unfortunately, it results in neglect of the other three senses.

Those three senses provide important information to the brain that your eyes and ears cannot pick up. For your mind to work at top efficiency, it has to receive clear, strong input from all your senses, all the time.

In order to keep all five senses sharp so they can continuously send clear signals to the brain, *you must use them.*

It is a great idea to deliberately strengthen your senses by going on sensory adventures. These adventures will keep all five senses sharp and will also help the brain create new neural connections as a result of receiving atypical sensory input. If you keep surprising the brain this way, it will have a reason to stay agile even at an advanced age.

A few examples of sensory adventures:

1. **Sense of smell**. Visit a flower shop. Go with a friend and take turns identifying flowers by their fragrance. Let your nose be your eyes.

2. **Sense of hearing.** Go to an active public place such as a park, or city square where there are benches. Sit with your eyes closed and listen to the sounds. What is happening? Paint a picture in your mind's eye about what your ears are 'seeing.'

3. **Sense of touch.** This is an easy one. Go to your closet (with your eyes closed, of course) and let your fingers be

your eyes. Feel the different fabrics – really feel them. See if you can 'see' and name the type of fabric just by touching it.

    a. In your mind describe each fabric as you touch it. Try tactile comparisons. Think about the differences in the tactile sensations between touching a fabric with your fingers vs. placing it against your cheek.

4. **Sense of taste.** The average person gulps down food without taking the time to really taste it. It is also common for people to only eat foods they know and like. That is a terrible waste of the sense of taste; however, it does provide some outstanding opportunities for sensory adventures.

    a. The next time you go grocery shopping, buy five or six small food items that are not included in your usual grocery list. Look for exotic and usual items that will be completely new to your taste buds.

    b. Taste the new foods like a professional. Bite off only a small amount and move it slowly around your mouth in order to explore the full flavor. Each part of the tongue detects a specific taste (i.e. bitter, sweet, etc.). You don't want to miss anything.

    c. Try each selection by itself, take your time, and discover the wonder of new taste sensations

5. **Sense of sight.** Although your eyes are used all the time, it does not mean that they have their fair share of productive stimulation. Visit a place that is filled with colorful items such as an arboretum, or even you own back yard when it is in bloom.

a. Flowering trees and plants are especially wonderful for this exercise. Take in all the shapes and colors of each plant. Study every detail. Notice the intricate, endless designs of nature and the wild array of shapes and colors.

These are only a few simple adventures, there are so many more. Try places like tide pools, a lakeside, the beach, the forest, the desert.

The possibilities are endless. Always be on the lookout for new and exciting ways to stimulate your brain by tickling your senses.

Put More Music in Your Life

Music is one of the oldest and most effective modes of therapy in the world. It has long been used to soothe children to sleep, and some research supports the theory that classical music can actually increase an unborn child's IQ.

Let's explore how it can contribute to a healthy brain and increase brain power in adults.

1. Music has been used effectively as a treatment for anxiety-related disorders. It would follow then, that it would also be effective in helping people to relax and let go of stress after a hard day.

2. Established studies have shown that music has the capacity to lower high blood pressure, and may also have a beneficial effect on patients suffering from dementia.

3. It has been found that listening to music and playing musical instruments can actually increase vital parts of the brain, like corpus callosum, which links the two hemispheres of the brain. When the both sides of the brain are working well and interactively, brain power is significantly increased.

4. Playing a musical instrument has also been shown to increase the size of the *motor cortex* of the brain. This is because playing an instrument requires not only knowledge and use of music theory; but, also requires dexterity and manual skill to play the instrument.

The conclusion is that whether you choose to play an instrument or listen to music, the benefits to the brain and your overall mental health are huge. In addition music can bring feelings of peace, happiness and great joy into your life.

This is a strategy that I encourage you to embrace wholeheartedly.

Making THINKING a Habit

The majority of people never learn to THINK and, in fact, they work very hard at avoiding it.

When faced with a problem, a project, or the need to make a decision, these undeveloped thinkers choose from a multitude of thinking avoidance tactics, for example:

1. They take action on the first thing that pops into their heads – no questions asked!

2. They ask *everyone* what they should do (including many people they shouldn't ask) and follow their advice, which is often very misguided.

3. They pick a solution from TV or a movie, forgetting that those situations are not real!

The mind is the greatest idea-generating machine that exists, and every person has complete, unrestricted access to his/her very own model; yet, rarely uses it effectively.

Your mind should always be your primary source for creative ideas, answers to questions, and solutions to problems.

The more your use your mind, the sharper it gets. The decline of mental acuity is not the result of ageing; it is the result of not being used. Practice THINKING every day!

Following is an adaptation of an exercise that I learned many years ago from Earl Nightingale in his classic tape series, *Lead the Field*. This series is still available today and I highly recommend it.

The exercise is so good that I wanted to share it with you in this book.

- Set aside 1 hour/5 days a week (early morning is good, but anytime will work).

- With a fresh cup of coffee, sit in a comfortable chair where you will be undisturbed.

- At the top of a blank sheet of paper, write the goal or topic you want to "think" about.

- Take a deep breath, relax and . . . let the mind go to work.

- List as many ideas as you can – shoot for a minimum of 10, 20 is better.

- Stay with it for 30 minutes to an hour – even if the ideas do not flow easily

Be warned – This kind of focused thinking will not be easy at first. It takes time to stimulate a brain that has become comfortable with not thinking, but once you get it going, you will be amazed at the results.

Remember *it takes at least 30 days to establish a habit.* This will be no different.

Now a word of caution! Most of the ideas each day will not be good. Let that be OK and keep going. Don't filter as you go. Remember, one good idea can be invaluable! Do not quit early even if the page remains blank. Regardless of the result each day, do it again the next day!

This can be a life-changing practice that will stimulate your brain and sharpen your mind every time you do it! It is time to become a THINKER.

Strategy Four: Expanding Horizons

Just as being a couch potato will eventually take its toll on your body, stagnation of the mind will also eventually take its toll. To live a full mentally active life that includes complete clarity of thought well into your 80's and 90's, continual brain stimulation is critical (as noted time and time again in this book). An incredibly fun way to stimulate your brain is by expanding your horizons in every way possible, beginning with . . .

Be Open to New Ideas

It is very easy to ignore the opinions of others, especially when they are significantly different from your own. Don't be afraid to find out more. Learning about different viewpoints does not mean that you have to agree with them.

It is also easy to walk away from new information or new ideas by rationalizing that you have too much going on right now to explore anything new.

One of the easiest and most exciting ways to stimulate your brain and expand your awareness is to be inquisitive about everything. Ask lots and lots of questions. Keep an open mind. Take every opportunity to learn everything you can – about EVERY thing.

Differences and varying viewpoints are what make life interesting and provide incredible stimulation for your brain. Processing unfamiliar perspectives and thoughts are a goldmine for the mind and create wonderful new pathways that expand your brain power.

You can even ask questions of yourself about a situation that is taking place near you, e.g. at another table in the food mall at your local shopping center.

For example: A guy hands a girl a small bouquet of roses. The girl takes the flowers, but doesn't make eye contact, and says nothing. The man also doesn't react to her seemingly indifference.

What kinds of questions would you ask about this situation if you were talking to someone else?

Important point: *You don't have to be involved* in a situation to ask the questions. You are simply stimulating your mind by wondering to yourself about what is going on. Ask as many questions as you can think of – then, try answering them. That is additional stimulation for the brain

Get in the habit of asking questions when you are watching TV or a movie. "Why did he do that?" "What happened to the other person?" "Who is really the bad guy in all of this? And what is his/her motive?"

A slightly different version of this exercise is to bring your imagination into the mix and make up a story about what is happening.

This is fun activity to do with a friend(s) when you are waiting for a movie to start, or when you are having coffee or dinner.

Try a Change of Scenery

There's a belief that humans are always searching for stability and safety – however, we also have this paradoxical need to see the world and experience the adventure of traveling to new places.

Never venturing far from home can put our brain in a rut and weaken your mental prowess. The mind stagnates and loses energy. Eventually you *will* feel stuck, and that will affect the way you feel about life in general.

Humans are not only social beings; everyone is born with a natural curiosity and spirit of adventure. If you don't believe me, just watch a young child explore his world.

It is thrilling to the human spirit to visit new places, to interact with people from different cultures (even within your own country). As we learn about other cultures, it spurs questions about ourselves and the place we call home. The entire experience provides an incredible push on the brain as it processes the new information.

In short, when embraced and enjoyed to its fullest, travel is a wonderful, exciting experience.

Traveling should not be considered a luxury – it should be considered a life imperative. It refreshes the mind, body, and spirit. It broadens your perspective, it creates wonderful memories that you can enjoy long after the trip has ended, and it makes you a more interesting person with things to talk about.

So – begin to plan your itinerary for this year's trip. Don't panic . . . you won't have to spend your life savings. There are amazing day trips and weekend trips that can be taken very close to home, within your own state, your own country and often within your own city.

Use the following questions to help make a list of "trips to be taken" and list them in a general order by possible dates.

1. Where have you always dreamed of going? Think of your top three. Are any of them realistic right now given your financial situation? If the answer is yes, pick a date and start to plan. If the answer is no, put it on your "to do" list for the future.

2. What historic landmarks in the country do you want to see? Why those particular ones? Are there any close to your home that could be a day or weekend trip? What kind of preparation (study) would you like to do before you go?

3. What are some trips that could be planned around your passions or hobbies? If you are interested in music, is there a particular city that you would like to visit because of its history and local culture? Are you a sports fan and have a particular ballpark you would like to visit – or maybe the Baseball Hall of Fame?

4. What is the one city in the U.S. that you would like to visit, and why? What is the one country in the world that you would like to visit, and why?

5. What adventures can you plan in your own city, the surrounding area or within the state?

6. Who are (or could be) your preferred traveling companion(s), or do you prefer to travel alone?

I encourage you to put this strategy on your list, even if it is just a daydream at this point. Being a seasoned traveler myself, I can tell you there is nothing that stretches and refreshes the mind and heart more that spending time in cultures different from your own.

Strategy Five: Introspection

Develop Self-Awareness

How well do you know yourself? Are you clear on your values, your priorities, your drivers, the story you tell yourself about what you can and cannot do?

Why is developing self-awareness an important strategy for increasing brain power? The answer is: If you are not willing to be introspective and find the answers to those questions, plus many others, you are running the risk of losing control of the way you think about yourself and about life.

The mind cannot decipher between truth and fiction. As a result, when you are carrying heavy loads of emotional baggage, continual negative thoughts, and false beliefs about yourself, your mind will act on that information as if it were all true.

The results are fairly predictable, for example: alienation from family, few close friends, low self-esteem, on-going mental anguish, and physical stress, when added together can lead to physical and/or mental illness.

When you are willing to make the effort to develop a clear sense of who you really are, you can develop tools to handle life's experiences very differently than when you are working from a void. BTW, who you really are, may be very different from what you tell yourself, or what others tell you,

You are less likely to be overly stressed when you have a deep understanding of your internal self. You recognize and accept your strengths and your weaknesses and are capable of developing tools to build on the first and succeed in spite of the second.

You can face life with much greater confidence because defeat and failure are not deep sinkholes that you must struggle to crawl out of. They become life lessons to be studied and absorbed. The newly gained wisdom will give you the confidence to move forward with greater insight into the human mind (including your own), and the world around you.

I hope you can see how the experiences that result from a deep self-awareness can be very stimulating for the mind and will contribute to better physical and mental health.

Motivate Yourself – Begin the Journey Today

Are you motivated to take this journey? I promise it will be a good one if you take it seriously and make a commitment to yourself to enjoy the ride.

Motivation is definitely an inside job. No one can motivate you to do anything that you do not have good personal reasons for doing. If you aren't motivated to do this, or any project for that matter, I guarantee the problem is that you do NOT have a good enough reason to move forward. That means that the first step before the journey begins is always to find a good reason for taking the journey.

A good reason is what you to go back to when the going gets rough. It keeps the mind focused and refuels the energy when it drops.

A good reason can be developed into a glorious picture of how the end of the journey will look. The picture should be so clear that it becomes a magnet that pulls you into the future.

The picture should include:
- Where you will be?
- How will you look?
- Who will be with you?
- How will you feel physically?
- How will you feel emotionally and mentally?
  (This one is a big one)

The clearer you can make the picture of your destination, the more powerful its pull will be.

The human brain is not capable of discerning between imagination and what's happening in reality. It is very much capable of accepting that which we imagine as reality. Make your preferred destination of this journey a reality.

Conclusion

There you have it! I hope you have enjoyed reading the five simple strategies and the individual action steps within each section. Once your personal action plan is implemented and the steps become a natural and free-flowing part of your lifestyle, they will contribute to a lifetime of brain power.

Hopefully, you have already completed Step 1: *Make Brain Power a Priority*, and also finished Step 2: *Read the Book.* Now it is time to complete Step 3: *Create an Action Plan.*

The choices within each strategy can be used with equal impact on the health of your brain and ongoing strength of your cognitive abilities. Some of the suggestions probably appealed to you more than others. I hope that you made note of those as you were reading.

You may have noticed that some of the suggested actions require more work than others. It would be wise to choose a few at first that can be easily incorporated into your lifestyle. This will give you a greater chance for success and will help build momentum. Small steps are always a good idea when making major changes.

After you are comfortable with your first few choices, add others, one at a time, until you have tried them all. You will eventually settle on the ones that work best for you – or, if you like them all, switch them out for variety!

As I said in the beginning, the one exception to "optional activities" is *The Basics*. All of the basics must be implemented if you are fully committed to improving your brain power; but, there are choices within each of the three basics – food selection, types of exercise, etc.

Use all the information in good health. ENJOY!

I would love to hear from you – your thoughts, ideas, and experiences with the strategies.

You can reach me at wilsonemarketing@gmail.com.

J. J. Jackson

References

Anderson, V. *7 Brain Boosters to Prevent Memory Loss*, Retrieved 23 Jan 2012 from **http://www.webmd.com/healthy-aging/features/7-brain-boosters-to-prevent-memory-loss**.

Anthes, E. (2008) *6 Ways to Boost Brain Power*. Retrieved 23 Jan 2012 from **http://www.staff.vu.edu.au/sokolov/Resume/Culture/SAMIND_BrainPower_V2a.pdf**.

Drew. *50 Ways to Boost Your Brain Power,* Retrieved 23 Jan 2012 from **http://4mind4life.com/blog/2008/02/06/50-ways-to-boost-your-brain-power/**.

Franklin Institute. *Journey of the Developing Brain.* Retrieved 23 Jan 2012 from **http://www.fi.edu/learn/brain/exercise.html#top**.

Gillman, S. *70 Ways to Increase Your Brain Power.* Excerpt from Chapter 5 of **A Book of Secrets**. Retrieved 23 Jan 2012 from **http://www.mindpowernews.com/BrainPower.htm**.

Gómez-Pinill, F. (July 2008) *Brain foods: the effects of nutrients on brain function.* Perspectives, Volume 9. Retrieved 23 Jan 2012 from **http://www.ibp.ucla.edu/research/gomezpinilla/publications/nrn2421.pdf**.

Good Food. (2012). *10 Foods to Boost Your Brain Power.* Retrieved 23 Jan 2012 from **http://www.bbcgoodfood.com/content/wellbeing/features/boost-brainpower/1/**.

Ingemann, M. *The Power of Mind Mapping.* Retrieved 23 Jan 2012 from **http://www.mapyourmind.com/ebook.pdf**.

Kozarenko, V. (2006). *GMS Manual: Real Memory Improvement.* Retrieved 15 Jan 2012 from **http://www.realmemoryimprovement.com/GMS_Manual_RMI.pdf**.

Litemind. (2012). *120 Ways to Boost Your Brain Power.* Retrieved 19 Jan 2012 from **http://litemind.com/boost-brain-power/**.
Medina, J. (29012) *Brain Rule Rundown.* Retrieved 23 Jan 2012 from **http://www.brainrules.net/exercise?scene=**.

Mountain State Centers for Independent Living. (2012). *Understanding and Dealing With Stress.* Retrieved 14 Feb 2012 from **http://www.mtstcil.org/skills/stress-deal-4.html**.

Nightingale, E. (1988). *Lead the Field.* Audio cassette recording. Nightingale- Conant Publishing. Wheeling, IL.

O'Brien, S. *How Speaking Two Languages Can Improve Your Brain.* Retrieved 14 Feb 2012 from **http://seniorliving.about.com/od/lifelonglearning/a/How-Speaking-Two-Languages-Can-Improve-Your-Brain.htm**.

Scott, E. (2007). *Top 8 Strategies to Sharpen Thinking Skills.* Retrieved 23 Jan 2012 from **http://stress.about.com/od/stresshealth/tp/thinking_skills.htm**.

Smith, M. & Robinson, L. (2012). *How to Improve Your Memory.* Retrieved 23 Jan 2012 from **http://www.helpguide.org/life/improving_memory.htm**.

Uscher, J. *6 Top Concentration Killers.* Retrieved 23 Jan 2012 from **http://www.webmd.com/balance/features/top-concentration-killers**

Web MD, 50+ Live Better, Longer. *Healthy Aging - Emotional and Mental Vitality.* Retrieved 23 Jan 2012 from **http://www.webmd.com/healthy-aging/tc/healthy-aging-emotional-and-mental-vitality?page=2**.

Wellsource, Inc. *Improve Your Memory.* Retrieved 23 Jan 2012 from **http://wellsource.info/wn/hc-memory.pdf**.

Willingham, D. T. *What Will Improve a Student's Memory?* American Educator: "Ask the Cognitive Scientist". Retrieved 23 Jan 2012 from **http://www.aft.org/pdfs/americaneducator/winter0809/willingham.pdf**.

www.ingramcontent.com/pod-product-compliance
Lightning Source LLC
Chambersburg PA
CBHW072339290526
45794CB00002B/945